Your Amazing Itty Bitty® Concussion Book

15 Things You Should Know About Brain Injuries

Sheryl Hensel

Published by Itty Bitty® Publishing
A subsidiary of S & P Productions, Inc.
Copyright © 2015 Sheryl Hensel

Printed in the United States of America

Itty Bitty® Publishing
311 Main Street, Suite E
El Segundo, CA 90245
(310) 640-8885

ISBN: 978-1931191166

I dedicate this book to my mother, Rae Hensel, who has always been there for me and supports me in all that I do. A woman couldn't ask for a better mother than you. I love you.

Also, for all of you who have had an injury to your head and never thought of it as a possible brain injury. You know the dots don't connect the same, but really don't know why. I hope this book helps connect some of the dots for you.

Stop by our Itty Bitty® website to find interesting blog entries regarding Brain Injury and Concussion.

www.IttyBittyPublishing.com

Or visit Sheryl Hensel at:

www.sherylhensel.com

Table of Contents

Step 1
Understanding the Brain

In this Itty Bitty® Book you will find 15 things to help you understand brain injuries. When an injury to the head occurs it's often overlooked as insignificant. Disruptions can occur physically, emotionally and of course, mentally. The most important things to know about the brain is:

1. It is divided into two hemispheres, right and left.
2. The right hemisphere controls the left side of the body and vice versa.
3. The lobes of the brain are: Frontal, Parietal, Occipital and Temporal.
4. The brain stem and Cerebellum are the other major parts of the brain.
5. The brain is a 3-pound organ with 100,000,000,000 (100 billion) brain cells!
6. The brain can process information at 268 mph.
7. 60% of your brain is fat.
8. Lack of oxygen in the brain for 5-10 minutes results in brain damage.
9. Neurons carry messages within the brain.
10. Performing certain exercises can physically increase your brain's strength, size and density.
11. When awake, a small light bulb can be powered by the electricity of the brain.

Functions of Each Region of the Brain

- Right Hemisphere: Artistic, Creative, Intuitive, Music Awareness, 3-D Forms
- Left Hemisphere: Academic, Logical, Analytic, Language, Reasoning, Written
- Frontal Lobe: Concentration, social and sexual behavior, judgment, attention span, impulse control, problem-solving, organization, critical thinking
- Parietal Lobe: Visual attention, touch, face recognition, understanding time, sensations, body awareness
- Temporal Lobe: Memory, new learning, hearing, understand spoken language, order, categorization, rhythm
- Occipital: Visual perception, hallucination, illusions, color recognition
- Brain Stem: Breathing, swallowing, heart rate, balance, sleep, alertness, Autonomic Nervous System
- Cerebellum: Coordination, balance, equilibrium

Step 2
What is a CONCUSSION?

It is an injury to the brain that often alters the way your brain functions. Most people recover quickly if the brain is given appropriate time to heal.

Concussions are usually the most basic injury to the brain. They can be mild or severe and the symptoms can often be subtle. Being equipped with some basic facts can help you determine what action needs to be taken.

1. Every concussion is unique.
2. A concussion is considered a traumatic brain injury (TBI).
3. It may take days, weeks, or months before realizing the brain was traumatized.
4. Not all people who experience a concussion lose consciousness.
5. Multiple concussions can cause the brain to have a longer recovery time.
6. NO jolt to the head should be considered insignificant.
7. The brain is resilient and if you need to relearn skills that were lost, it can be done.
8. A learning disability may be a TBI from an early life incident needing brain rehab.

Tips: Dealing with Concussions

Sometimes the signs are very obvious, but often they go unnoticed. What you may "hear," but not "see," is the following:

- "I just don't feel like myself"
- "I'm so tired and don't know why"
- "Things just aren't clicking"

If you suspect that somebody has had a concussion, don't let them just "sleep it off."

- Awaken the injured person every three-four hours to evaluate changes in symptoms.
- Have them state what day it is and their name.
- No drug or alcohol use after a concussion.
- Rest is important, but not total bed rest.
- Limit activities that require thinking.
- Graduated return to play. Start with aerobic and resistance exercises to test their limits.
- Consult a doctor regarding any drug use.

There is no need to flash a light in their eyes after a concussion. The brain needs rest, so having downtime can accelerate their recovery.

Step 3
You Might Not Think These Cause a Brain Injury

Some of the items listed below might surprise you, because some are everyday occurrences. Not all concussions come from a MAJOR slam to the head that results in a coma or amnesia. This is a brief list that may "jolt your memory" of an incident that may have caused a TBI.

1. Being born
2. Shaken as a baby
3. Learning to walk and hitting your head on objects e.g., tables, floor, stairs
4. Cheerleading & gymnastics stunts
5. Falls: thrown from a horse, falling off a bicycle, intoxicated events, icy slips, skiing
6. Traffic accidents & forceful whiplash
7. Assaults or domestic violence
8. Struck by or against: standing up with a cupboard above your head, roller coasters
9. Active duty in military war zone
10. Sporting activity e.g., football, boxing, soccer
11. Viruses and parasites
12. Studies find long-term mobile phone use increases the risk of brain tumors

Tips: Critical Consideration

By listing the previous activities, I don't want you to think in any way I'm suggesting to not participate in them. Live life and have fun; just be aware that some hang-ups, OCD, memory issues, etc., you have today may stem from a head trauma that occurred YEARS ago.

What I do want you to contemplate from the previous list is:

- The brain **is** resilient and can heal itself.
- The brain sits on a little stem surrounded by fluid. No outside padding can totally protect your brain from slamming against the inside of your skull.
- A helmet can definitely help protect you somewhat from the severity of injury.
- With every concussion you experience, the more detrimental it can be to your brain health...ESPECIALLY IN A SHORT AMOUNT OF TIME BETWEEN CONCUSSIONS!
- Blood vessels may stretch.
- Cranial nerves may be damaged.
- A blood clot in the brain could occur and be fatal.

Step 4
Types of Brain Injuries

1. **Traumatic Brain Injury** (TBI)
   a. Concussion
   b. Contusion – a bruise (bleeding) on the brain
   c. Coup-Contrecoup – both sides of brain hit the skull
      ~ front/back
      ~ side/side
   d. Diffuse Axonal – caused by shaking or strong rotating force
      ~ Shaken Baby Syndrome
      ~ Causes brain structures to tear and chemicals to be released
   e. Penetration – gunshot, knife, sharp object
2. **Acquired Brain Injury** (ABI)
   Caused by:
   a. Degenerative disease
   b. Tumors
   c. Strokes
   d. Cancers
   e. Toxins
   f. Near drowning
   g. Anoxia (brain not getting any oxygen)
   h. Hypoxia (brain gets some oxygen but not enough)

Levels of Brain Injury

The levels of brain injury are "scored" by the **Glasglow Coma Scale (GCS).** GCS is a neurological scale that attempts to give a reliable, objective way of recording the conscious state of a patient. There are initial and subsequent assessments administered which measure improvements or deterioration of the person's condition.

- Mild TBI
  - GCS score 13-15
  - May or may not lose consciousness
  - Testing or scans may appear normal

- Moderate TBI
  - GCS score 9-12
  - Loss of consciousness from a few minutes to a few hours

- Severe Brain Injury
  - Usually requires radical treatment
  - Often open head injuries, but can also be closed head injuries

Step 5
Signs and Symptoms

While every concussion is not the same, there are commonalities amongst brain injuries. They may be subtle signs and not immediately apparent.

1. **Physical Signs**
   a. Headache
   b. Nausea and/or vomiting
   c. Balance and visual problems
2. **Cognitive/Mental Signs**
   a. Slow reaction and delayed responses
   b. Trouble concentrating
   c. Trouble remembering
3. **Emotional Signs**
   a. More emotional
   b. Sadness/Depression
   c. Irritability
4. **Sleep**
   a. Sleeping more or less than usual
   b. Drowsiness or trouble falling asleep

People who go to the ER with head trauma are often monitored and released without guidance of any kind.

Be proactive when you start finding yourself making compensations for your deficits, particularly as they apply to cognitive signs.

Signs/Symptoms (cont.)

- **More Physical signs**
  - Dizziness and fatigue
  - Slurred speech
  - Sensitivity to light and noise
  - Tingling/Numbness
  - Experiences seizures
  - Convulsions
  - Ringing in the ears
- **More Cognitive/Mental signs**
  - Trouble recognizing people
  - "Foggy" brain
  - Trouble recalling recent conversations or information
  - Repeating questions
- **More Emotional Signs**
  - Quick tempered
  - Nervousness
  - Changes in personality

Step 6
Long-Term Effects and When to Seek Medical Help

Ignoring the early symptoms of a concussion and delaying treatment can lead to longer recovery time and can be life threatening. Multiple impacts to your skull put you at higher risk of long-term cognitive impairment. The movie *Concussion* has shed some light on the importance of early treatment. These possible outcomes are not worth thinking it's "just a bump to my head." Bumps on the head can cause:

1. Epilepsy
2. Seizures
3. Increased risk of Alzheimer's and Parkinson's disease
4. Early on-set dementia
5. Hormone deficiencies
6. Concentration and memory problems
7. Sensory issues with smell, taste and vision
8. Emotional and behavioral problems
9. Premature death

The severity of the impact, frequency of blunt force trauma, and their subsequent treatment, will make a big difference in the long-term effects.

Is It Time for 911?

When in doubt, it's best to play it safe and seek medical assistance. If you're uncertain, one or more of the following will be a good guideline.

- Vomiting
- Losing consciousness temporarily
- Loss of coordination
- Severe headache
- Slow pulse and/or slowed breathing
- Feeling over stimulated by light and noise
- Not remembering the accident
- Slurred speech
- Weakness or numbness
- Can't be awakened
- One pupil (black part of eye) is larger than the other
- Clear fluid or blood coming from the nose, ears or mouth
- Loss of bowel or bladder control

The signs for children are the same, but also include not being able to be consoled, don't want to eat and won't stop crying.

Step 7
Statistics

According to the CDC, 2002 – 2006

1. An estimated 1.7 million people sustain TBI annually. Of those:
   a. 52,000 die
   b. 275,000 are hospitalized
   c. 1.365 million, nearly 80%, are treated and released from ERs
2. TBI is a contributing factor to one-third (30.5%) of all U.S. injury-related deaths.
3. About 75% of TBIs that occur each year are concussions or other forms of mild traumatic brain injury (MTBI).
4. Direct medical costs and indirect costs of TBI, such as lost productivity, totaled an estimated $60 billion in the United States in 2000.
5. Once every 3 minutes a child goes to ER due to a sports-related concussion.
6. Concussion rates doubled from 2005-2012 in U.S. high school athletes.
7. Every 7 minutes someone dies from a brain injury.
8. Lifetime cost for a survivor of a severe brain injury is estimated to exceed $4 million.
9. 1 million children sustain a brain injury each year.

TBI Statistics

- Unfortunately, at the present time, the Center for Disease Control and Prevention website posts their most current statistical information only through 2010.
- Every 23 seconds, one person in the U.S. sustains a brain injury.
- The increase of TBI's, and the impact it has on overall health and workplace productivity, is draining – physically, emotionally and financially.

Step 8
What to Say and/or Do to Help

If someone you know and love has had a TBI, the support and understanding you give can make a huge difference in their rehabilitation.

1. Try to be compassionate and think of the person as if they had a cast on their brain. How would you treat them if you SAW the injury?
2. Just like in the movie, *50 First Dates,* make accommodations to help them rather than be frustrated over what has happened to them. Get the entire family on board with a plan to help.
3. Life has changed for them and things just aren't the same. The simplest tasks can be daunting and they can't remember what they know they should remember.
4. The person you knew is gone; celebrate and discover the person they are becoming.
5. Please understand – they aren't lazy or stupid, but they are healing; you just can't see it.
6. What they do and why they do it doesn't make sense to them or to you. Just think, "Oh yeah, it's their brain thing."

Helpful Hints

- Acknowledge their injury without pity.
- Establish routines together until things are familiar.
- Put important dates in their phone calendar for them.
- In the beginning, keep multiple conversations in a room to a minimum.
- When you see a confused look on their face, slow down and circle back around the discussion without being obvious.
- Understand that behavior problems might be an indication of an inability to cope.
- Patience, patience, patience.
- Listen without trying to solve their problems.
- Learn all you can about TBI's.
- Sticky notes are a blessing.
- Manage your expectations of them.
- Don't take things personally that they say or do. Understand it's a "brain" thing.

Helpful Phrases

- "I don't know what you're going through but I'm here to help if you need it."
- "Good job."
- "What can I do to help?"

Step 9
What NOT to Say and/or Do

Let's just make it easier on everybody and *forget the "WHY" statements*. They probably just don't know and if they did, they might not be able to explain "it."

1. Sympathetic people may say, "Oh, everybody has memory lapse" or "It's part of the aging process." That devalues what a person is going through.
2. If you test them to see how they are doing, you will most likely be disappointed. Just know things aren't the same and don't expect them to be the same.
3. It helps if you don't patronize them or talk to them like they're a child. Sometimes the confused look on their face is their brain processing the information. They aren't being difficult – they are just trying to dive deep in the memory well.
4. Getting upset at them over an emotional outburst is pointless. They're probably already beating themselves up and trying to figure out why they did that.

Verbal Danger Zones

- "Don't you remember when--____?"
- "We just talked about this yesterday."
- "How many times do I have to tell you?"
- "Why do you sleep all of the time?"
- "Why are you looking at me like that?"
- "You never used to be like (or do) that."
- "When will things get back to normal?"
- "I know what you're going through."
- "You LOOK fine."
- "Maybe if you tried harder."
- "You sure are grumpy."
- "Let me do that for you."
- "Stop being so negative."
- "You're lucky to be alive."
- "I want the old you back again."

A note to the concussion victim:

I wish I could tell you all of your family and friends will be supportive and there for you. That often isn't the case because they just don't understand. You LOOK like the same "old you," but you don't ACT like the same "old you." Rather than try to understand your sometimes irrational behavior, it's just easier to leave the friendship. Just know you aren't alone in that scenario.

Step 10
Brain Rehabilitation and Services

A great deal of cognitive rehabilitation is done on the computer. When you feel tired, doctors suggest looking out the window at something far away and green. It relaxes the brain.

Here are some other ideas:

1. Draw or copy shapes
2. Take mentally challenging classes: quilting or digital photography
3. Play Iota: A desktop card game
4. Play computer games like Awesome Memory
5. Use iphone apps like Corkulous Pro
6. Use the Lumosity: Brain-Training App
7. Use puzzle books and jigsaw puzzles
8. Stimulate your mind with artistic pursuits, craft and social activities
9. Intermittent fasting
10. Be sure to get enough sleep. 7-9 hours is important for brain detoxification. Sleep loss results in the loss of neurons.
11. Take Progesterone (female hormone)

Types of Therapy

The therapy needed will depend on which area of
the brain was damaged. The following is a partial
list of common therapies people with TBI seek
out to address the isolated symptoms of the
condition. They may be helpful, but they don't
address the root causes of the problem – TBI.

- Speech: communication skills
- Optometrist: visual impairment
- Cognitive: perception, memory, thinking
- Audiologist: hearing and balance
- Physical: restore motor function
- Respiratory: breathing difficulty
- Occupational: daily living & work skills
- Recreational: social skills
- Sexual: speaks for itself ☺
- Behavioral: behavior modification

If you have had a head injury, you must treat the
brain and not the symptoms. If you know you
have had a head injury and you are exhibiting
many of the symptoms listed in this book,
mention the fact to your primary care physician.
Ask if the head injury could be related to the
problems. Brain injury treatment is still in its
early stages of development. Be proactive if you
suspect a TBI.

Step 11
Natural Remedies & Aids

The following are some suggestions for alternative TBI therapies:

1. Quantum Energetics Structural Therapy (QEST)
2. Craniosacral Therapy
3. Hyperbaric Oxygen Treatment
4. Neurofeedback
   a. In which electrodes are hooked to the scalp and the patient is trained to speed up brain activity
5. Meditation:
   a. Harvard study shows this rebuilds the brain's grey matter in 8 weeks
6. Acupuncture
7. Chiropractic therapy
8. Massage
9. Vitamin D and Omega 3 (animal based)
10. Opposite Exercise
    a. Come up with 10 words and think of the opposite word
11. Light Therapy (LED)
    a. Boosts the output of nitric oxide near LEDs placement, improves blood flow to the brain

Natural Alternatives (Cont.)

- **Exercises**: Grow and expand the brain's memory center 1-2% per year
  - High-intensity interval
  - Strength training (super slow)
  - Stretching and core work
  - Walking 10,000 steps a day
  - Yoga
  - Aerobic exercise
- **Healthy foods suggested by Dr. Mercola**
  - Curry, walnuts, pecans, macadamia nuts, red meat, blueberries, crab, salmon, avocado
  - Krill oil and coconut oil
  - Fresh vegetables (i.e., celery, broccoli, cauliflower)
  - Garbanzo beans (chickpeas)
  - **NOT so helpful** – sugar and grain carbohydrates
- **Essential Oils: Increase oxygen to the brain:**
  - Veiver, Patchouli, Cedarwood, Sandalwood, and Frankincense
- **Essential Oils blend that calm and ease panic attacks:**
  - Frankincense, Chamomile, Romane, Lavender, Bergamot, and Mandarin

Step 12
What Coaches Need To Know

These action steps are based on recommendations presented in the International Concussion Consensus Statement.

1.   Educate: coaches, parents and athletes
2.   Remove an athlete from play who is believed to have a concussion – **right away**.
3.   Obtain permission to "return to play." An athlete can only return to play or practice after at least 24 hours, with permission from a health care professional.
4.   There is NO concussion-proof helmet, but it IS recommended a helmet be worn to prevent a concussion from becoming a serious brain injury.
5.   The brain is like an egg toss. The yolk is the brain, the egg white is cerebral spinal fluid, and the shell is skull. Every time the egg is tossed, the yolk rebounds off the shell. That is much like an impacted brain to the skull.

Coaches Need to Know

- A concussion can happen without losing consciousness.
- Helmets need to be properly fitted and well-maintained.
- Acute Concussion Evaluation (ACE) is a cognitive test.
- There's a training program available to non-medical professionals – the Certified Brain Injury Specialist – which is offered through the Academy of Certified Brain Injury Specialists.
- Have a <u>Return to Play</u> protocol that is progressive before allowing full-time play.
- Develop a parent packet to educate the caretaker.
- 50% of "second impact syndrome" incidents – brain injury caused from a premature return to activity after suffering the initial injury (concussion) – result in death.
- Emergency room visits for concussions sustained during organized team sports doubled among 8-13 year olds between 1997 and 2007, and nearly tripled among older youth.

http://nfhslearn.com/ Heads Up by CDC for concussion training

Step 13
For The Caregiver

Severe TBI causes your life to suffer a drastic change as your loved one is no longer the same person.

1. Create a circle of care to help you with the new requirements needed.
2. Seek out friends, neighbors and paid caregivers; just make sure you're all on the same page. DON'T try to go it alone.
3. Attend support groups! It can be too hard to endure the combination of:
   a. losing the person you once knew
   b. prolonged stress
   c. physical demands of caregiving
   d. the biological vulnerabilities that come with age, which place you at risk for significant health problems, as well as an earlier death.
4. Take care of yourself first and don't feel guilty when you take the time you need and ask for help.

Caregivers are more likely to have a chronic illness than are non-caregivers, namely:
- high cholesterol
- high blood pressure
- obesity
- depression

Resources

The following are some good books, journals, websites and authorities.

- Dr. Perlmutter's *New York Times* best-selling book, _Grain Brain_.
- "The English Surgeon" documentary details Neurosurgeon Henry Marsh's fascinating career.
- _Reclaim Your Brain: Revolutionary New Book_ by Daniel Amen, M.D.
- www.quantumenergeticshealing.com
- www.mercola.com
- www.davidwolfe.com
- http://danielamenmd.amenclinics.com
- www.caregiver.org/traumatic-brain-injury
- www.biausa.org
- Health Resources and Services Administration. Maternal and Child Health does have grants available. Visit www.mchb.hrsa.gov
- *"Concussion,"* the informative movie, starring Will Smith as Dr. Bennet Omalu.

Step 14
Military and Brain Injuries

According to the Veterans Administration (*November 18, 2014),* traumatic brain injury has become the hallmark injury of a generation of veterans, following more than 13 years of war in Iraq and Afghanistan.

1. Between 2000 and July 2012, more than 253,000 service members sustained a TBI. Common causes of TBI include explosive devices, falls and vehicle or motorcycle accidents.
2. Concussions and Post Traumatic Stress Disorder (PTSD) are thought to be "cousins." It is believed that if one is left untreated, treatment for the other often stays stalled.
3. "The perfect storm." When PTSD and TBI coexist, it's often difficult to sort out what's going on. One feeds and reinforces the other.
4. The parts of the brain damaged in PTSD:
   a. Frontal lobe which houses our emotions
   b. Amygdala which oversees our fight or flight response

Support for Veterans

Beginning in 2007, the VA implemented mandatory TBI screening for veterans getting care in VA; specifically, those who served in combat operations and separated from active duty service after September 11, 2001.

- The Defense and Veterans Brain Injury Center's (DVBIC) TBI Recovery Support Program, formerly known as the Regional Care Coordination Program, provides services and resources to:
    - military members
    - members of the National Guard and reserves
    - veterans who have sustained a TBI
    - family members and caregivers
- http://dvbic.dcoe.mil/about/tbi-military
- Depending on the extent of the injury, vets are eligible for up to 100% disability rating. If you are a military veteran with a service-related disability, you may qualify for compensation ranging from $133 to more than $3,300 in monthly benefits.
- http://www.brainlinemilitary.org/

Step 15
Final Thoughts: Your New "Normal"

Your brain injury is like NO OTHER. No one can say that they know what you're going through. What can be said is:

1. Your brain can heal.
2. With 99% certainty, you will lose a friend and probably a family member because they don't understand the "new you."
3. Your brain possesses the ability to:
   a. reorganize pathways
   b. create new connections
   c. create new neurons throughout your entire lifetime
4. In my own experience, Quantum Energetics Structural Therapy (QEST) allowed my body to heal my TBI.
5. Neuroplasticity or brain plasticity— means you are reforming your brain with each passing day.
6. Seek out the medical care that will help you heal.
7. Research which healing process works best for you.
8. Find a support a group that is uplifting and solution-oriented – not a pity party of complainers.

Final Thoughts on TBI

- The brain sits on top of a stem and is surround by fluid and protected by a skull.
- There is no "wrapping" around the brain – just the fluid.
- Keep the visual in your mind from the movie "*Concussion.*" A glass jar filled with fluid and an object. Shake that jar (your skull) and the fluid (cerebral spinal fluid) will slosh around and your brain (object in jar) will hit the walls of the jar.
- Two brain injuries in close succession can kill.
- Will Boggs, M.D. states, "While most trauma centers have policies in place that reflect current guidelines for treating severe TBI, most follow those guidelines in less than 75% of patients.
- Many NFL players leaving the sport suffer from chronic traumatic encephalopathy, or CTE, a degenerative disease.
- CTE occurs when repetitive head trauma begins to produce abnormal proteins in the brain. The proteins work to form tangles around the brain's blood vessels, interrupting normal functioning and eventually killing nerve cells themselves.

You've finished. Before you go...

<u>Tweet/share that you finished this book.</u>

Please star rate this book.

Reviews are solid gold to writers. Please take a few minutes to give us some itty bitty feedback.

ABOUT THE AUTHOR

I'm not a medical professional, nor do I write this Itty Bitty® book from a Western Medical agenda. I'm a survivor of a brain injury and hope to impart information to you in the simplest terms, yet in a very understandable way about what I have learned as a result of my injury.

I began my career as a middle school teacher, where I was drawn to the service of children and learning. I was on top of my game and recently promoted to a new position as the district-wide School-to-Work Coordinator. My path, however, took an entirely new direction two years later in 1998.

Waiting at a stoplight I witnessed a car veer across traffic and crash onto the sidewalk, luckily not striking anybody. I rushed to assist the driver, and moments later while speaking with 911, I was struck by another motorist. I sustained a severe closed head injury and brain trauma. Despite extensive rehabilitation and western medicine treatment, I continued to suffer from migraines, limited cognitive functioning, general pain and depression.

The hardest part of it all was that I "looked" okay, but things just weren't clicking inside. It's frustrating to know you don't remember things like you used to and visibly you appear to be fine. Unlike a casted leg where people can SEE the injury, a closed head trauma is invisible to most, sometimes even the person who suffers from one. The day after my accident a student brought a gun to the school where I taught and killed himself minutes before classes started.

God knew that was one experience I didn't need to carry with me through life. On that day, I was very grateful for the accident that happened just the day before.

While living and teaching full time in Florida, I flew to Colorado every six weeks to learn the powerful healing work of QEST. Frankly, I couldn't afford to make these trips on a teacher's salary. However, I couldn't afford NOT to make them, and I didn't know why.

A year after starting classes, my mother was diagnosed with Stage 4 cancer. Ten years later, after many QEST sessions, mom is cancer-free and takes ZERO medication.

Today I am a QEST practitioner! This scientific healing method corrects physical symptoms and emotional traumas at the root cause. This powerful work has helped restore physical, emotional and spiritual health and create new vitality for clients with TBI, cancer, migraines, depression, and a myriad of other conditions (minor and major), where traditional approaches have failed. *QEST work all started with brain injuries and progressed from there.*

If you enjoyed this book you might also enjoy…

Your Amazing Itty Bitty® Cancer Book –
Jacqueline Kreple

**Your Amazing Itty Bitty® Self-Esteem
Book** – Jade Elizabeth

**Your Amazing Itty Bitty® Marijuana
Manual** – Kat Bohnsack

And many more Itty Bitty® Books available in
paperback and on the digital sites.